36 Meal Recipes for People Who Have Had a Loss of Appetite:

All Natural Foods Packed With Nutrients to Help You Increase Hunger and Improve Appetite

By

Joe Correa CSN

COPYRIGHT

This publication is designed to provide accurate and authoritative information in regard to the subject matter covered. It is sold with the understanding that neither the author nor the publisher is engaged in rendering medical advice. If medical advice or assistance is needed, consult with a doctor. This book is considered a guide and should not be used in any way detrimental to your health. Consult with a physician before starting this nutritional plan to make sure it's right for you.

ACKNOWLEDGEMENTS

This book is dedicated to my friends and family that have had mild or serious illnesses so that you may find a solution and make the necessary changes in your life.

36 Meal Recipes for People Who Have Had a Loss of Appetite:

All Natural Foods Packed With Nutrients to Help You Increase Hunger and Improve Appetite

By

Joe Correa CSN

CONTENTS

ABOUT THE AUTHOR

After years of Research, I honestly believe in the positive effects that proper nutrition can have over the body and mind. My knowledge and experience has helped me live healthier throughout the years and which I have shared with family and friends. The more you know about eating and drinking healthier, the sooner you will want to change your life and eating habits.

Nutrition is a key part in the process of being healthy and living longer so get started today. The first step is the most important and the most significant.

INTRODUCTION

36 Meal Recipes for People Who Have Had a Loss of Appetite: All Natural Foods Packed With Nutrients to Help You Increase Hunger and Improve Appetite

By Joe Correa CSN

Loss of appetite is a very common issue and a first step and cause to various diseases. Insufficient intake of healthy nutrients weakens the immune system and that's the critical moment when we start to get exposed to different bacterias, viruses, etc.

Poor nutrition, lack of physical activity, and medications are the most common reasons for loss of appetite.

From my own experience, I have created these delicious recipes that helped me boost my own appetite and have a balanced diet full of nutrients.

By combining good nutrition with 30 minutes of excercise every day, you will see results fast. This book offers some great old-fashioned and classic recipes with some simple tricks to make them more appealing and enjoyable, while keeping them reasonably easy to prepare.

A good trick to increase your appetite is to try to make your food look good which will make it more enticing to eat.

This book offers lots of different recipes to increase your appetite and to eat with the same delight everyday.

Bon Appetit!

36 MEAL RECIPES FOR PEOPLE WHO HAVE HAD A LOSS OF APPETITE: ALL NATURAL FOODS PACKED WITH NUTRIENTS TO HELP YOU INCREASE HUNGER AND IMPROVE APPETITE

1. Cheddar Cheese Casserole

Ingredients:

4 free range eggs

1 cup of cheddar cheese, crumbled

1 bell pepper, chopped

1 medium-sized onion, sliced

2 large potatoes, shredded

½ tsp of salt

½ tsp of black pepper, ground

1 tbsp of olive oil

1 tsp of parsley

Preparation:

Preheat the oven to 370°F.

Heat up the oil over in a large frying skillet over a medium-high temperature. Add the onion and stir-fry for 1 minute.

Now, add potatoes and pepper. Cook for about 5 minutes, or until potatoes nicely crisp. Stir constantly. Remove from the heat and transfer to a baking dish.

Pour the eggs over and add crumbled cheese. Reduce the temperature to low and bake for 20 minutes or until doneness. Remove from the oven and sprinkle with fresh parsley. Set aside to cool.

Serve.

Nutrition information per serving: Kcal: 292, Protein: 17.5g, Carbs: 5.8g, Fats: 1.4g

2. Orange Cranberry Smoothie

Ingredients:

¼ cup of orange juice

¼ cup of cranberries

½ cup of Greek yogurt

¼ cup of skim milk

1 tbsp of chia seeds

1 tsp of fresh mint, minced

Preparation:

Combine all in a blender. Blend until smooth and transfer to a large serving glasses. Top with fresh mint and refrigerate at least 1 hour before serving.

Enjoy!

Nutrition information per serving: Kcal: 326, Protein: 13.1g, Carbs: 32.4g, Fats: 10.6g

3. Cornflour Chicken Breasts

Ingredients:

2 chicken breasts, boneless, skinless, and thinly sliced

2 cups of cornflour

2 medium-sized tomatoes, chopped

3 garlic cloves, minced

1 large egg

1 tsp of vegetable seasoning mix

½ tsp of black pepper, ground

½ tsp of Cayenne pepper, ground

1 tbsp of vegetable oil

1 tbsp of sour cream

Preparation:

Preheat the oven to 400°F.

Combine cornflour, tomato, garlic, cayenne pepper and vegetable seasoning mix in a food processor. Blend until smooth mixture. Set aside.

Whisk the egg in a bowl. Dip the meat in egg, and place to large greased baking sheet. Pour the blended mixture over and coat well with a spoon.

Bake for 20 minutes, or until chicken fork-tender. Remove from the heat and set aside to cool. Top with sour cream for some extra taste.

Nutrition information per serving: Kcal: 244, Protein: 25.3g, Carbs: 22.8g, Fats: 5.7g

4. Peach & Blueberries Parfait

Ingredients:

1 large peach, chopped

½ cup of sour cream

1 cup of blueberries

1 tbsp of honey

1 tbsp of almonds, finely chopped

Preparation:

Layer the ingredients as listed. Repeat layers until full glasses.

Drizzle with pomegranate seeds on top.

Refrigerate for 30 minutes before serving.

Nutrition information per serving: Kcal: 310, Protein: 12.4g, Carbs: 43.2g, Fats: 7.7g

5. Spicy Rice and Broccoli

Ingredients

2 cups of white rice, long-grain

1 lb of broccoli, halved

1 cup of button mushrooms, chopped

1/2 cup of sweet cream

1 cup of cottage cheese, shredded

½ tsp od salt

2 tbsp of olive oil

½ tsp of red pepper flakes

Preparation:

Preheat the oven to 370°F.

Cook the rice using package instructions. Drain and set aside.

Combine mushrooms, sweet cream and a pinch of salt in food processor. Blend until creamy mixture. Set aside.

Gently, place the broccoli in a boiling water and cook for 5 minutes. Remove from the heat and drain well.

Grease a baking sheet with oil. Spread the rice equally over. Now add broccoli and spread over the rice.

Spoon mushroom cream on top. Bake for 40 minutes. remove from the oven and cut into cubes for serving. Drizzle with cheese and red pepper flakes.

Nutrition information per serving: Kcal: 293, Protein: 17.4g, Carbs: 42.7g, Fats: 8.7g

6. Mexican Turkey Patties

Ingredients:

1 lb of ground turkey

½ cup of apple cider vinegar

¼ tsp of garlic, minced

¼ tsp of cumin, ground

1 tsp od fresh coriander, finely chopped

¼ tsp of chili pepper, ground

1 tbsp of vegetable oil

Preparation:

Combine all ingredients in a large bowl. Stir all well to combine. Using your hands, form the patties.

Heat up the oil in a large frying pan over a medium-high temperature. Gently place the patties using a spatula. Cook for about 10 minutes on each side.

Remove from the heat and drain with paper towels.

Serve with some fresh vegetable salad or yogurt.

You can freeze the mixture and use it later as well.

Nutrition information per serving: Kcal: 104, Protein: 16.8g, Carbs: 41.3g, Fats: 11.7g

7. Beet & Blueberries Smoothie

Ingredients:

1 medium-sized beet, chopped

¼ cup of blueberries, frozen

¼ cup of vanilla yogurt

1 tsp of lemon juice

1 tsp of lemon zest

1 tbsp of honey, raw

Preparation:

Combine beet, blueberries, vanilla yogurt, honey, and lemon juice in a food processor. Blend until smooth.

Top with lemon zest and blueberries for extra taste. Refrigerate for 1 hour before serving.

Nutrition information per serving: Kcal: 119, Protein: 4.2g, Carbs: 14.5g, Fats: 5.3g

8. Mozzarella Toast

Ingredients:

2 garlic clove, minced

2 tbsp of olive oil

1 tsp of fresh parsley, finely chopped

3 oz of Mozzarella cheese, sliced

4 bread slices, toasted

Preparation:

Place the bread slices in the toaster and set to light brown. Using a kitchen brush, spread the oil over the bread slices. Make a fine layer of cheese and sprinkle with a pinch of fresh parsley.

You can add tomato slices or lettuce leaf for some extra taste. This is, however, optional.

Nutrition information per serving: Kcal: 142, Protein: 6.3g, Carbs: 6.5g, Fats: 4.3g

9. Banana Pancakes

Ingredients:

1 large banana, pureed

1 cup of all-purpose flour

2 free-range eggs

1 tbsp of honey

1 tbsp of baking powder

1 cup of skim milk

2 tbsp of vegetable oil

Preparation:

Combine flour, banana, baking powder and honey in a large mixing bowl. Stir well to combine.

In a separate bowl, whisk the eggs, milk and 1 tablespoon of oil. Now, pour this mixture into the flour bowl. Use a hand mixer to make a nice lumpy batter.

Heat up 1 tablespoon of oil in a frying pan over a medium-high temperature.

Now pour about ¼ cup of batter onto the pan and cook until browned, and then flip over with a wide spatula.

Repeat the process until done.

Serve pancakes with honey or some fresh fruits by your choice.

Nutrition information per serving: Kcal: 235, Protein: 7.2g, Carbs: 48.2g, Fats: 5.3g

10. Eggs & Green Onions Soup

Ingredients:

4 cups of chicken broth

2 large eggs

2 egg whites

1 cup of green onions, chopped

1 garlic clove, minced

1 tsp of salt

½ tsp of black pepper, ground

2 large potatoes, peeled and cut into bite-sized pieces

1 medium-sized carrot, sliced

1 tsp of cornstarch

1 cup of green onions

1 tsp of finely chopped parsley

Preparation:

Pour the vegetable broth into a deep pot over a medium-high temperature. Bring it to a boil and remove from the heat. Set aside.

In a separate pot, combine potatoes and carrot . Add a pinch of salt and bring cook for about 10 minutes, or until potatoes are fork-tender. Remove from the heat and drain well. Transfer to the vegetable broth.

Whisk the eggs and egg whites properly and stir it in the pot. Add remaining spices and cover with a lid. Reduce the temperature to low, and cook for 15 minutes.

Nutrition information per serving: Kcal: 325, Protein: 21.7g, Carbs: 47.2g, Fats: 7.3g

11. Marinated Trout

Ingredients:

2 lbs of trout, cleaned

2 large potatoes, peeled and cut into wedges

For the marinade:

3 tbsp of olive oil

3 garlic cloves, crushed

1 tbsp of fresh rosemary, finely chopped

1 tsp of white pepper, crushed

1 tsp of dried thyme, ground

1 tsp of salt

3 bay leaves

Preparation:

Combine marinade ingredients in a large baking sheet. Set aside.

Wash and pat dry the fish. Place it into the marinade and coat well. Refrigerate for one hour.

Preheat the oven to 400°F.

Add potato wedges and bake for 25 to 30 minutes, or until fish is fork-tender. Serve with lemon slices.

Nutrition information per serving: Kcal: 279, Protein: 24.6g, Carbs: 56.7g, Fats: 14.8g

12. Asian Chicken Salad

Ingredients:

1 lb of chicken breasts, pre-cooked, cut into bite-sized pieces

1 cup of spring onions, chopped

1 cup of celery, chopped

½ cup of fresh parsley, finely chopped

1 tsp of fresh coriander, finely chopped

2 cups of Romaine lettuce, chopped

For dressing:

1 tbsp of balsamic vinegar

2 tbsp of orange juice

1 tsp of salt

1 tbsp of vegetable oil

1 tsp of sesame seeds

1 tsp of almond, roughly chopped

¼ tsp of black pepper, ground

Preparation:

Combine all ingredients except chicken, in a large bowl. Stir once and set aside.

Combine all dressing ingredients in a mixing bowl. Stir well and set aside to allow flavors to meld for about 10 minutes.

Drizzle the dressing over the vegetables and top with chicken chops. Sprinkle with pepper for extra taste.

Nutrition information per serving: Kcal: 246, Protein: 24.6g, Carbs: 98.7g, Fats: 10.3g

13. Sweet Veal Steaks

Ingredients:

1 lb of veal steaks, boneless, thinly sliced

1 orange, peeled and cut into wedges

½ of small lemon, peeled

1 tbsp of yellow mustard

1 tbsp of honey

2 tbsp of balsamic vinegar

½ tsp of salt

½ tsp of black pepper, ground

1 tbsp of basil, finely chopped

Preparation:

Preheat the oven to 400°F.

Combine orange, lemon, mustard, honey, and vinegar in a food processor. Blend until smooth and set aside.

Place the steaks in a large baking sheet. Pour the mixture over and sprinkle with salt and pepper.

Bake for 45 to 50 minutes, or until doneness. Remove from the oven and serve with fresh basil.

Nutrition information per serving: Kcal: 121, Protein: 16.2g, Carbs: 12.3g, Fats: 5.6g

14. Couscous Tomato Salad

Ingredients:

3 large tomatoes, diced

1 cup of couscous

½ cup of Mozzarella cheese, diced

2 tbsp of fresh spring onions, finely chopped

2 tbsp of olive oil

1 tbsp of lemon juice

1 garlic clove, crushed

¼ tsp of black pepper, ground

1 tsp of fresh basil, finely chopped

1 cup of water

½ tsp of red pepper flakes

Preparation:

Combine tomatoes, cheese, lemon juice, spring onions, olive oil, garlic, salt, and pepper in a mixing bowl. Cover with a lid and refrigerate. Marinate for about 30 minutes to allow flavors to meld.

Pour water into a large frying saucepan and bring it to a boil. Stir in the couscous and remove from the heat immediately. Cover with a lid and set aside for 5 minutes. Stir few times.

Now, combine tomato and cheese mixture with drained couscous in a serving bowl. Stir in the basil and toss well properly.

Sprinkle with red pepper flakes for some extra taste and serve.

Nutrition information per serving: Kcal: 142, Protein: 5.8g, Carbs: 28.4g, Fats: 6.3g

15. Ziti Beef

Ingredients:

1 lb of beef steak, chopped into bite-sized pieces

2 small onions, sliced

1 large bell pepper, chopped

1 medium-sized zucchini, peeled and cubed

1 cup of tomato sauce

½ tsp of salt

½ tsp of black pepper, crushed

1 tsp of fresh parsley, finely chopped

Preparation:

Preheat the oil in a slow cooker over a medium-high temperature. Add the onions and saute until translucent.

Add meat chops,bell pepper, and zucchini. Sprinkle with some salt and pepper to taste. Stir well to combine.

Seal the lid and reduce the temperature to low. Cook for about 20 minutes, and remove from the heat. Let it stay for 15 minutes, and then open the lid.

Meanwhile, follow the package instructions to cook ziti pasta. Drain well and transfer to a serving plate.

Stir in the beef into the pasta and serve. Top with some fresh parsley.

Serve warm.

Nutrition information per serving: Kcal: 121, Protein: 16.2g, Carbs: 12.3g, Fats: 5.6g

16. Cabbage Soup

Ingredients:

1 lb of cabbage, shredded

1 cup of celery, chopped

4 medium-sized carrots, sliced

2 garlic cloves, crushed

2 large tomatoes, chopped

1 medium-sized onion, chopped

½ tsp of salt

1 tsp of vegetable seasoning mix

1 cup of vegetable broth

3 cups of water

Preparation:

Combine tomatoes and onions in a blender well until smooth.

Meanwhile, combine all other ingredients in a slow cooker. Add the tomato and onion mixture and stir well.

Cover with lid and cook for 4 hours over a medium-high temperature.

Nutrition information per serving: Kcal: 87, Protein: 2.4g, Carbs: 17.2g, Fats: 6.4g

17. Red Peppers with Goat's Cheese

Ingredients:

1 cup of Goat's cheese, crumbled

2 large bell peppers, seeded and cut into strips

2 garlic cloves, minced

1 small onion, sliced

1 tbsp of olive oil

1 tbsp of honey

1 tbsp of apple cider vinegar

1 tsp of dried basil, minced

2 lettuce leaves, whole

½ tsp of salt

¼ tsp of black pepper, ground

Preparation:

Preheat the oil in a large frying skillet over a medium-high temperature. Add onions and garlic and stir-fry until translucent. Add peppers and cook for about 10 minutes, or until fork-tender.

Stir in honey, vinegar, basil, salt, and pepper. Cook for 5 more minutes stirring occasionally. Remove from the heat and let it cool for few minutes.

Line lettuce leaves on a serving plate. Transfer the peppers and sauce onto lettuce leaves, and top with cheese.

Nutrition information per serving: Kcal: 165, Protein: 6.5g, Carbs: 4.8g, Fats: 14.3g

18. Guava Mango Smoothie

Ingredients:

1 medium sized mango, peeled and chopped

1 medium-sized guava, peeled and chopped

½ cup of Greek yogurt

¼ cup of skim milk

1 tbsp of honey

1 tbsp of whipped cream

1 tsp of cocoa, raw

Preparation:

Combine mango, guava, yogurt, milk, and honey in a food processor. Blend until smooth. Transfer to a serving glasses and top with whipped cream. Sprinkle with cocoa for extra taste!

Nutrition information per serving: Kcal: 115, Protein: 4.1g, Carbs: 24.5g, Fats: 1.2g

19. Spinach & Cheddar Cheese Salad

Ingredients:

5 oz of baby spinach, finely chopped

½ cup of cheddar cheese, crumbled

1 large apple, shredded

For the dressing:

1 tbsp of balsamic vinegar

3 tbsp of extra-virgin olive oil

1 tbsp of Dijon mustard

1 tsp of cumin, ground

1 tsp of vegetable seasoning mix

1 tbsp of water

½ tsp od salt

½ tsp of black pepper, ground

Preparation:

Combine all dressing ingredients in a mixing bowl. Stir well to combine and set aside.

Combine baby spinach and shredded apple in a large serving bowl. Top with cheese. Drizzle with marinade and give a good stir. Set aside for a few minutes to allow flavors to mingle.

Serve immediately.

Nutrition information per serving: Kcal: 420, Protein: 8.2g, Carbs: 15.8g, Fats: 21.6g

20. Quinoa Chili Stew

Ingredients:

8 oz of button mushrooms, sliced

1 cup of kidney beans, pre-cooked, drained and rinsed

½ lb of chicken breasts, skinless and boneless, cut into bite-sized pieces

1 cup of quinoa, pre-cooked

½ cup of cottage cheese, shredded

1 small chili pepper, chopped

½ tsp of dried oregano, ground

½ tsp of cumin, ground

1 cup of tomato sauce

3 cups of chicken broth, unsalted

½ tsp of fresh coriander, finely chopped

1 cup of water

Preparation:

Place mushrooms and water in a large frying skillet over a medium-low temperature. Cover with a lid and cook for 10 minutes, or until fork-tender. Remove from the heat and set aside.

Combine kidney beans, oregano, cumin, and chili in a food processor. Blend until smooth and transfer to the mushroom skillet. Pour the chicken broth and add chicken chops and tomato sauce.

Add quinoa and coriander. Give it a good stir to combine. Cover with a lid and cook for 20 minutes. Remove from the heat and stir in the cheese. Set aside for few minutes to cool.

Top with fresh coriander and serve warm.

Nutrition information per serving: Kcal: 210, Protein: 17.8g, Carbs: 32.4g, Fats: 5.7g

21. Raisins and Carrot Salad

Ingredients:

1 cup of raisins, chopped

5 medium sized carrots, sliced

1 cup of spring onions, chopped

¼ cup of almonds, roughly chopped

For the dressing:

2 tbsp of lemon juice

2 tbsp of olive oil

½ tsp of curry powder

1 tbsp of maple syrup

Preparation:

Combine all dressing ingredients in a mixing bowl. Stir all well to combine and set aside.

Now combine all salad ingredients in a medium serving bowl and drizzle with dressing. Serve immediately.

Nutrition information per serving: Kcal: 219, Protein: 4.7g, Carbs: 27.8g, Fats: 3.2g

22. Salmon Green Omelet

Ingredients:

6 free-range eggs

4 oz of wild smoked salmon, skinless, boneless, and cubed

¼ cup of asparagus, chopped

1 garlic clove, crushed

1 tsp of fresh dill, minced

1 small onion, sliced

1 tsp of lemon juice

1 tbsp of olive oil

2 tbsp of fresh parsley, finely chopped

1 tbsp of skim milk

½ tsp of salt

¼ tsp of black pepper, ground

Preparation:

Beat the eggs in mixing bowl. Add milk, dill, parsley, salt, and pepper. Whisk well to combine and set aside.

Meanwhile, heat up the oil in a large frying skillet over a medium-high temperature. Add garlic and onions. Stir-fry for 5 minutes, or until translucent. Add asparagus and lemon juice. Cook for 4-5 minutes stirring occasionally.

Add the eggs mixture and cook for 3-4 minutes and flip the omelet. Now add salmon chops, and cook for 2 minutes more. Remove from the heat and serve warm.

Nutrition information per serving: Kcal: 169, Protein: 12.5g, Carbs: 5.3g, Fats: 10.3g

23. Oatmeal Smoothie

Ingredients:

½ cup of oatmeal

½ cup of Greek yogurt

1 tbsp of honey

½ cup of fresh strawberries, halved

1 tbsp of quinoa

Preparation:

Combine all ingredients in a blender. Blend until smooth and transfer to a serving glass. Top with quinoa for some extra nutrients!

Refrigerate for 30 minutes before serving.

Nutrition information per serving: Kcal: 212, Protein: 19.8g, Carbs: 33.6g, Fats: 1.8g

24. Black & White Soup

Ingredients:

5 oz of white beans

5 oz of black beans

2 medium-sized red onions, minced

1 medium-sized carrot, sliced

4 oz of Brussel sprouts, halved

2 garlic cloves, finely chopped

5 cups of chicken broth, (or vegetable broth for vegetarians)

½ tsp of black pepper, ground

½ tsp of sea salt

1 tbsp of vegetable oil

Preparation:

Place beans and lentils in a large pot. Pour enough water to cover all and bring it to a boil over a high temperature. Remove from the heat and let it soak in the water for about 1 hour. Drain well and set aside.

Meanwhile, heat up the oil in a deep pot over a medium-high temperature. Add onions and stir-fry for few minutes, until translucent. Add Brussel sprouts and carrot. Cook for about two minutes, stirring occasionally. Now, pour in 5 cups of chicken broth, and add pre-cooked beans and lentils. Adjust the thickness of the soup with broth. Add a pinch of salt and pepper to taste.

Reduce the temperature to low, and cover with a lid. Cook for about 45 minutes. Remove from the heat and let it cool a little bit.

Sprinkle with some fresh parsley. This is, however, optional.

Nutrition information per serving: Kcal: 179, Protein: 11.3g, Carbs: 31.7g, Fats: 15.4g

25. Warm Peach and Cranberries Porridge

Ingredients:

½ cup of dried peaches, chopped

½ cup of dried cranberries, chopped

1 tbsp of flaxseeds

¼ cup of skim milk (or coconut milk)

1 tbsp of honey

1 tsp of vanilla extract

1 tsp cocoa, raw

Preparation:

Combine peaches, cranberries, and flaxseeds in a medium pot. Pour water to cover all ingredients. Bring it to a boil and reduce the heat to low. Add milk and cook for 2 minutes more. Remove from the heat and stir in the honey and vanilla.

Transfer to a serving bowl and sprinkle with cocoa for extra taste.

Nutrition information per serving: Kcal: 258, Protein: 2.6g, Carbs: 51.4g, Fats: 10.2g

26. Portobello Mushroom Burgers

Ingredients:

5oz Portobello mushrooms

¼ cup of extra virgin olive oil

2 garlic cloves, crushed

½ tsp of dried oregano, crushed

1 tbsp of parsley, finely chopped

¼ tsp of sea salt

¼ tsp of freshly ground black pepper

3 tbsp of mayonnaise

2 tbsp of cheddar, grated

1 large onion, finely chopped

Preparation:

In a medium-sized bowl, whisk together olive oil, garlic, oregano, parsley, salt, and pepper. Using a kitchen brush, spread the mixture over each mushroom and set aside for 20 minutes.

In another bowl, combine mayonnaise with cheddar and chopped onion. You can add some more salt to taste, but this is optional. Use the mixture to stuff each mushroom.

Preheat the grill pan over medium-high heat. Place the mushrooms, top side up and cook for about 7 minutes, or until lightly charred.

Nutrition information per serving: Kcal: 204, Protein: 10.5g, Carbs: 12.2g, Fats: 15.7g

27. Chicken Scallopini in a Creamy Sauce

Ingredients:

2 chicken breast halves, boneless and skinless

¼ cup of butter

1 garlic clove, crushed

1 tsp of dry oregano

¼ cup of fresh lime juice

1 cup of button mushrooms, sliced

½ cup of Gorgonzola cheese, chopped

1 cup of sour cream

3 tbsp of Parmesan cheese, grated

½ tsp of salt

½ cup of all-purpose flour

1 tbsp of honey

½ cup of wine

Preparation:

In a small bowl, combine the flour with sour cream, butter, honey, Parmesan cheese, and Gorgonzola. Add fresh lime juice and beat well with electric mixer, on high.

Season each chicken breast half with salt and oregano. Place in a slow cooker. Add the creamy mixture, wine, mushrooms, and garlic.

Cover the pressure cooker and set on low for 6-7 hours.

Useful tip:

You can replace wine with fresh orange juice for sweet taste.

Nutrition information per serving: Kcal: 273, Protein: 45.3g, Carbs: 9.4g, Fats: 4.8g

28. Almond and Vanilla Smoothie

Ingredients:

½ cup of coconut milk

2 large eggs

1 tbsp of coconut oil

1 tbsp of almonds, minced

1 tsp of pure vanilla extract, sugar-free

½ cup of water

½ tsp of stevia

Preparation:

Place the ingredients in a blender and pulse to combine. Serve cold.

Nutrition information per serving: Kcal: 498 Protein: 31g, Carbs: 5g , Fats: 40g

29. Broccoli and Beef Pasta Bake

Ingredients:

14 oz of lean ground beef

17oz of dried pasta

12 oz of broccoli, sliced

½ cup tomato paste

1 tsp dry oregano, ground

½ tsp of salt

¼ cup butter, melted

1 tbsp of olive oil

½ cup of Cheddar cheese, grated

Preparation:

Combine the tomato paste with oregano, and melted butter. Stir well.

Heat up the olive oil over a medium-high heat. Add ground beef, season with some salt, and cook until brown, stirring constantly. Remove from the heat. Place sliced broccoli at the bottom of your slow cooker. Then add dried pasta, ground beef, and tomato paste mixture.

Cover and set on low for 4-6 hours, or until pasta is tender. Remove from the heat and spread the grated Cheddar. Cover again and allow the cheese to melt.

Serve warm.

Serving tip:

Top with sour cream or Greek yogurt.

Nutrition information per serving: Kcal: 327, Protein: 13.6g, Carbs: 42.5g, Fats: 12.5g

30. Mango porridge

Ingredients:

1 medium-sized mango, chopped

1 medium-sized pineapple, chopped

½ cup of butter

2 tbsp of coconut flakes

2 cups of crackers, crushed

1 tsp of honey

Preparation:

Preheat the oven to 375°F.

Combine crushed crackers, honey, and coconut flakes in a mixing bowl.

Melt butter in a frying pan and stir it in the crackers mixture. Stir all well to combine. Set aside.

Place the mango and pineapple chops into a large baking dish. Spread the crackers mixture over the fruits equally. Place it in the oven and bake for 25 minutes, or until fork-tender. Remove from the oven and let it cool for a while.

Top with ice cream ball.

Nutrition information per serving: Kcal: 251, Protein: 8.4g, Carbs: 42.6g, Fats: 7.3g

31. Beef Stroganoff

Ingredients:

2 lbs of stew beef

1 oz of butter

2 large onions, finely chopped

1 garlic clove, crushed

1 cup of button mushrooms, sliced

½ cup of Gorgonzola, crumbled

1 ½ cup of sour cream

½ tsp of salt

½ tsp of black pepper, ground

¼ cup of water

3 cups of rice, pre-cooked

Preparation:

Combine the ingredients, except the sour cream, in a slow cooker. Cover and set on low for 8 hours.

If you set the heat on high, you can reduce the cooking time to 5 hours.

When done, stir in sour cream and serve.

Nutrition information per serving: Kcal: 292, Protein: 20.6g, Carbs: 41.2g, Fats: 6.2g

32. Creamy Cheese Avocado

Ingredients:

1 ripe avocado

1 large tomato, finely chopped

1 large onion, peeled and finely chopped

2 tbsp of extra virgin olive oil

2 tbsp of tomato paste, sugar-free

¼ cup of cheddar cheese, shredded

1 tbsp of fresh lime juice

½ tsp of salt

1 tsp of cayenne pepper

Preparation:

Preheat the oven to 350°F. Line some baking paper over a baking sheet and set aside.

Slice the avocado in half and remove the stone. Using a sharp knife, cut criss-cross patterns to allow the spices to penetrate the avocado flesh.

In a medium-sized skillet, heat up the olive oil over medium-high heat. Stir-fry the onion for 2-3 minutes, or until translucent, and add chopped tomato. Continue to cook until fork tender. Now add tomato paste, fresh lime juice, salt, and cayenne pepper. Give it a final stir and remove from the heat.

Fill each avocado half with this mixture and top with cheddar. Bake for 20 minutes.

Nutrition information per serving: Kcal: 410 Protein: 1.4g, Carbs: 9.4g , Fats: 2.6g

33. Cherry Spinach Smoothie

Ingredients:

½ cup of cherries, frozen or fresh, pit removed

¼ cup of spinach, chopped

1 medium-sized banana, sliced

½ cup of almond milk

1 tbsp of honey

Preparation:

Place the ingredients in a blender and pulse to combine. Serve with some ice cubes.

Nutrition information per serving: Kcal: 58 Protein: 1.4g, Carbs: 9.4g , Fats: 2.6g

34. Cauliflower Macaroni with Italian Garlic Sauce

Ingredients:

6 cups of cauliflower florets

3 large ripe tomatoes

3 tbsp of extra virgin olive oil

2 garlic cloves, crushed

½ tsp of dry oregano

¼ tsp of salt

¼ cup of fresh lime juice

½ cup of coconut flour

1 cup of vegetable broth

Preparation:

Preheat the oven to 350 degrees.

Place cauliflower in a deep pot and add enough water to cover. Boil until done. Remove from the heat and drain. Set aside.

Whisk together vegetable broth with coconut flour. Set aside.

Peel and roughly chop the tomatoes. Make sure you keep all the liquid.

Heat up the olive oil over a medium temperature. Add the garlic and stir-fry for several minutes. Now add tomatoes, oregano, and salt. Reduce the heat to low and cook until the tomatoes have softened. Add lime juice and cook for 10 more minutes stirring constantly. Turn off the heat, add cauliflower and cover.

Let it stand for 10 minutes and transfer to a lightly greased baking sheet. Evenly pour over the vegetable broth.

Bake for 15-20 minutes or until you get a nice color on top.

Nutrition information per serving: Kcal: 293, Protein: 12.5g, Carbs: 9g, Fats: 3.99g

35. Choco-Coco Smoothie

Ingredients:

1 large egg

1 tbsp of coconut oil

1 tsp of chia seeds

¼ cup coconut milk

½ cup of water

1 tsp of stevia

1 tbsp of raw cocoa, sugar-free

½ tsp of vanilla extract, sugar-free

Preparation:

Place the ingredients in a blender and pulse to combine. Serve cold.

Nutrition information per serving: Kcal: 293, Protein: 12.5g, Carbs: 9g, Fats: 3.99g

36. Hot Vege Pizza Stuffed Peppers

Ingredients:

3 large green bell peppers

2 large tomatoes, roughly chopped

2 tbsp of tomato pizza sauce, sugar-free

1 tsp of dried oregano

½ tsp of thyme

4oz Mozzarella cheese, sliced

3 tbsp of parmesan cheese

1 tbsp parsley, finely chopped

4 tbsp of extra virgin olive oil

½ tsp of salt

¼ tsp of black pepper, freshly ground

Preparation:

Preheat the oven to 350 degrees. Line some baking paper over a baking sheet and set aside.

Using a sharp knife, cut the peppers in half and remove the seeds. Grease each paper inside with some olive oil. Set aside.

In a medium-sized bowl, combine mozzarella with tomatoes, pizza tomato sauce, thyme, oregano, parsley, and two tablespoons of olive oil. Stir well and use the mixture to stuff each pepper half. Add some salt and pepper and top with parmesan.

Bake for 20 minutes.

Nutrition information per serving: Kcal: 205, Protein: 11g, Carbs: 5g, Fats: 12g

ADDITIONAL TITLES FROM THIS AUTHOR

70 Effective Meal Recipes to Prevent and Solve Being Overweight: Burn Fat Fast by Using Proper Dieting and Smart Nutrition

By

Joe Correa CSN

48 Acne Solving Meal Recipes: The Fast and Natural Path to Fixing Your Acne Problems in Less Than 10 Days!

By

Joe Correa CSN

41 Alzheimer's Preventing Meal Recipes: Reduce or Eliminate Your Alzheimer's Condition in 30 Days or Less!

By

Joe Correa CSN

70 Effective Breast Cancer Meal Recipes: Prevent and Fight Breast Cancer with Smart Nutrition and Powerful Foods

By

Joe Correa CSN

www.ingramcontent.com/pod-product-compliance
Lightning Source LLC
Chambersburg PA
CBHW062152020426
42334CB00020B/2578